Mediterranean Diet Cookbook
for Chronic Kidney Disease

Your Guide to Renal Tasty and Nutritious Recipes, Elevate your well-being through the art of low-sodium, low-phosphorus, low-potassium diets with 14-Days Meal Plan and Easy 5 Mediterranean Friendly Exercises.

Cynthia P. Allison

About the Author

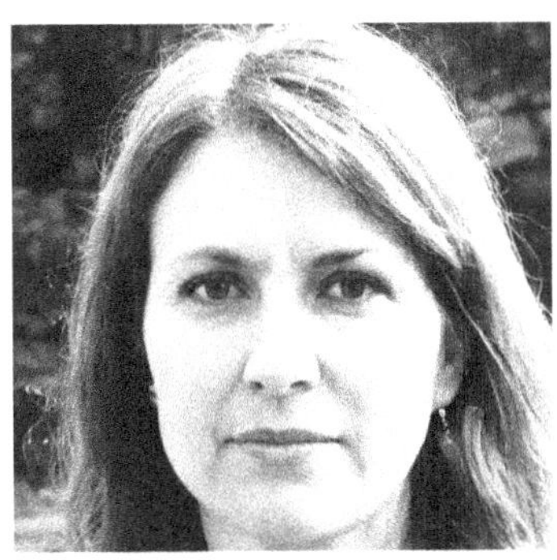Cynthia P. Allison, the creative force behind this insightful cookbook, is a seasoned writer with a passion for exploring the intersection of health and culinary arts. With a background in nutrition and a keen interest in the Mediterranean lifestyle, Cynthia has dedicated her writing to empower individuals managing chronic kidney disease.

Her expertise goes beyond words on paper; Cynthia is committed to delivering practical solutions and inspiring a mindful approach to eating. Drawing from real-life experiences and a genuine commitment to well-being, she shares not only delicious recipes but a holistic perspective on achieving kidney health through the lens of the Mediterranean diet.

Cynthia P. Allison represents the amalgamation of knowledge, creativity, and a genuine desire to make a positive impact on the lives of her readers. Join Cynthia on this culinary journey, where health meets flavor, and discover the transformative power of the Mediterranean diet for chronic kidney disease.

Explore, savor, and thrive with Cynthia P. Allison.

Table of contents

Introduction

Understanding the Mediterranean Diet for Kidney Health

Revealing the core principles

Renal health promotion and nutrition go hand in hand with the Mediterranean diet, which is well known for its heart-healthy advantages. This diet's main focus is on eating a lot of fruits, vegetables, whole grains, legumes, and healthy fats, with olive oil being a mainstay. It is essential to include lean protein sources like fish and chicken and to avoid consuming too much red meat, which has been linked to adverse effects on kidney function.

Most importantly, cutting back on salt is a key component of the Mediterranean diet, which is important for those with chronic renal disease. If people prefer using herbs and spices to add taste instead of too much salt, they may still enjoy food while protecting their kidneys.

The diet's intrinsic nutritional richness is a result of its base consisting mostly of whole, unprocessed foods. Significant potential for kidney protection can be found in the amount of antioxidants and anti-inflammatory substances present in fruits and vegetables. All these components work together to lower inflammation and oxidative stress, which can worsen kidney problems.

Furthermore, wine drinking in moderation and mindfulness are encouraged by the Mediterranean diet, especially when it comes to red wine. Although consuming large amounts of alcohol can be harmful to renal health, infrequent and moderate consumption of red wine may have positive effects on the cardiovascular system, supporting the diet's overall health-promoting message.

Essentially, the Mediterranean diet promotes a well-rounded, nutrient-dense, and palatable way of eating, which acts as a model for renal health. It offers people with chronic renal disease a sustainable and pleasurable way to maintain their overall health and well-being because of its emphasis on whole foods, careful protein selection, and conscious salt reduction. Applying the Mediterranean diet's tenets to daily life not only promotes gastronomic enjoyment but also turns into a proactive measure to protect and maintain renal function.

Examining the benefits for kidney wellness

Investigating the benefits of the Mediterranean diet uncovers a wealth of benefits that are especially beneficial for renal health. The diet has a strong focus on heart-healthy fats, such as those in olive oil. Olive oil, being high in monounsaturated fats, has been linked to better kidney function, decreased blood pressure, and decreased inflammation—all of which are crucial for preserving the best possible health of the kidneys.

Rich in vitamins, minerals, and antioxidants, the diet's profusion of fruits and vegetables is essential for maintaining renal function as a whole. These meals are rich in nutrients and help to reduce inflammation and oxidative stress, which supports a healthy renal environment.

An additional layer of kidney-friendly advantages is added to the Mediterranean diet by including lean protein sources like fish. The anti-inflammatory qualities of omega-3 fatty acids, which are abundant in fatty fish such as salmon, may lessen the strain on the kidneys and promote a stronger and more effective kidney system.

Utilizing herbs and spices sparingly rather than using a lot of salt is consistent with the diet's goal of lowering sodium consumption. By decreasing the load on the kidneys associated with digesting excessive levels of salt, the Mediterranean approach actively aids patients in controlling chronic kidney disease.

Additionally, the diet's emphasis on staying hydrated by drinking water and herbal teas is beneficial to kidney function. Maintaining a delicate balance that is critical for general health requires the kidneys to filter waste and poisons from the circulation, which they can only do with proper hydration.

The Mediterranean diet has advantages that go beyond health as a holistic way of living. Savoring tasty, nutrient-rich foods has psychological and emotional benefits that lower stress, which is proven to have a good effect on kidney function.

To put it simply, the Mediterranean diet is a multipurpose ally in the fight for kidney health. In addition to meeting the unique requirements of those with chronic renal disease, its well-considered blend of healthful, nutritious ingredients promotes an all-encompassing health philosophy that is in harmony with both taste and physiology.

Essential Ingredients and Cooking Techniques

The secret to opening up a world of tasty, nutrient-dense options is to understand the fundamental components and cooking methods of the Mediterranean diet for renal health.

1. **Extra virgin olive** oil is a mainstay in Mediterranean cuisine and is sometimes referred to as its heart. Its monounsaturated fats promote renal well-being and provide a healthy substitute for saturated fats. Use it for sautéing, drizzling, and dressing.

2. **Ample Fruits and Vegetables:** Indulge in a vibrant assortment of fresh produce, including berries, tomatoes, bell peppers, and leafy greens. They improve flavor and nutritional value because they are full of vitamins, minerals, and antioxidants.

3. **Whole Grains:** Choose whole wheat pasta, bulgur, and quinoa among other whole grains. These grains offer a tasty basis for many Mediterranean meals, as well as important nutrients and fiber.

4. **Lean Proteins:** When choosing protein sources, give priority to fish, poultry, lentils, and nuts. Without the added saturated fats that certain red meats have, these choices provide a nutrient-rich balance that supports kidney function.

5. **Herbs and Spices:** Elevate your recipes with a Mediterranean flair with herbs like basil, oregano, and thyme. Accept flavors that come from using cumin and garlic instead of too much salt.

6. Blow Your Energy on Seafood: Include high-oleic seafood, such as mackerel and salmon, that are high in omega-3 fatty acids. These good fats support kidney health because they have anti-inflammatory qualities.

Cooking Techniques

Cooking on the grill or roasting: Add a delicious smokiness to your food by grilling or roasting veggies and lean meats.

Mediterranean Salads: Make colorful salads by combining a variety of fresh vegetables. To add richness and healthy fats, use dressings made with olive oil.

Fish poaching and vegetable steaming are effective ways to retain nutrients. These low-heat cooking techniques preserve the nutritional value of foods.

One-Pot Wonders: Combine different ingredients to make nutritious, delectable meals with the least amount of cleaning possible. One-pot recipes simplify dinner preparation.

Nutty Finishes: When adding nuts, such as walnuts or almonds, to meals or toppings, you may impart a richness of taste and crunch.

Mindful Portion management: To ensure that your diet is balanced, practice mindful portion management. Accept the Mediterranean diet's emphasis on quality over quantity and relish every mouthful for optimum health.

Choosing kidney-friendly staples

Choosing foods that are good for your kidneys is a crucial part of following the Mediterranean diet for kidney health. So let's examine the fundamental components that underpin a healthful and kidney-conscious food adventure:

1. Low-potassium Vegetables: Give veggies like bell peppers, cabbage, and cauliflower priority since they have a lower potassium level. These nourish the body with vital nutrients without taxing the kidneys excessively.

2. Apples and Berries: Choose fruits with lower potassium content, such as apples and berries, to add sweetness to your meals without raising your potassium levels too much.

3. White Bread and Pasta: To control your consumption of phosphorus, go with white bread and pasta instead of whole grains. This choice preserves essential carbs while adhering to a kidney-friendly philosophy.

4. Egg Whites: Use egg whites as a source of protein in your diet. They provide an excellent source of protein without the phosphorus that is present in egg yolks.

5. Olive Oil as the Main Source of Fat: Adopt olive oil as your cooking's main source of fat. Its monounsaturated fats are in line with kidney-conscious options and offer a heart-healthy alternative.

6. Skinless Poultry: Stick to skinless poultry, such as turkey or chicken. With a high level of nutrients and little phosphorus, this lean protein source is kind to the kidneys.

7. **Low-Phosphorus Dairy substitutes:** Go for rice or almond milk as low-phosphorus dairy substitutes. These solutions don't add a lot of phosphorus while yet maintaining the creamy texture in recipes.

8. **Fresh Herbs and Spices:** Add flavorful herbs and spices, like cinnamon, cilantro, and basil, to dishes. These taste great and don't include any extra phosphorus or potassium.

9. **Cauliflower Rice:** Try using cauliflower rice as a kidney-friendly alternative to regular rice to control your phosphorus consumption while still getting a tasty and diverse food.

10. **Limit Sodium with Fresh Ingredients:** Use herbs and spices as seasonings and concentrate on utilizing fresh ingredients to lower your blood sodium levels. Reducing the consumption of processed and high-sodium meals is essential for renal health.

By knowing your way around these kidney-friendly mainstays, you can make a varied and filling Mediterranean-inspired dinner that is specifically designed with renal health in mind. You may maintain ideal kidney function and have a tasty and health-conscious eating experience by making thoughtful decisions.

Chapter 1

Breakfast Recipes

Mediterranean Avocado Toast with Tomato and Feta

Preparation Time: 10 minutes   *Total Time: 10 minutes*   *Servings: 2*

Ingredients:

- 2 ripe avocados
- 4 slices of whole grain bread
- 1 large tomato, sliced
- 1/2 cup crumbled feta cheese
- Fresh basil leaves for garnish
- Olive oil for drizzling
- Salt and pepper to taste
- Optional: Lemon juice for added freshness

Instructions:

1. Mash the ripe avocados until smooth in a basin.
2. For extra freshness, add a dash of optional lemon juice along with salt and pepper for seasoning.
3. Toast the pieces of whole-grain bread until they reach the desired crispness.
4. On each toasted piece of bread, equally distribute the mashed avocado.
5. Arrange fresh tomato slices over the avocado mixture.
6. Drizzle the tomato slices with feta cheese crumbles.
7. Add some fresh basil leaves as a garnish to each toast to enhance its taste and appearance.

8. Finally, drizzle a little olive oil over the toasts that have been put together. Present and Savor

Nutritional Value (Per Serving):

Calories: 250 kcal.	Protein: 8g.	Fat: 18g
Carbohydrates: 15g.	Fiber: 7g.	Sugar: 2g

Greek Yogurt Parfait with Berries and Almonds

Preparation Time: 5 minutes   *Total Time: 5 minutes*   *Servings: 2*

Ingredients:

- 2 cups Greek yogurt
- 1 cup mixed berries (strawberries, blueberries, raspberries)
- 1/4 cup almonds, chopped
- Honey for drizzling

Instructions:

1. Layer Greek yogurt with a mixture of berries in serving dishes or glasses.
2. Then top the berries with chopped almonds.
3. Drizzle with honey.
4. Layers may be repeated as needed.
5. Enjoy this tasty Greek yogurt parfait right away by serving it.

Nutritional Value (Per Serving):

Calories: 300 kcal.	Protein: 20g.	Fat: 15g
Carbohydrates: 25g.	Fiber: 5g.	Sugar: 15g

Quinoa Breakfast Bowl with Spinach and Poached Egg

Preparation Time: 15 minutes　　　*Total Time: 20 minutes*　　　*Servings: 2*

Ingredients:
- 1 cup cooked quinoa
- 1 cup fresh spinach, chopped
- 2 poached eggs
- Cherry tomatoes, sliced
- Avocado slices
- Feta cheese crumbles
- Olive oil for drizzling
- Salt and pepper to taste

Instructions:
1. Put the cooked quinoa and chopped spinach in a bowl.
2. Spoon into dishes with the combination of quinoa and spinach.
3. Add feta cheese crumbles, avocado, cherry tomato, and poached egg pieces to the top of each bowl.
4. Add a drizzle of olive oil and season with pepper and salt.
5. Serve immediately for a healthful Quinoa Breakfast Bowl.

Nutritional Value (Per Serving):

Calories: 350 kcal.　　　Protein: 18g.　　　Fat: 15g

Carbohydrates: 35g.　　　Fiber: 6g.　　　Sugar: 2g

Mediterranean Omelette with Spinach, Tomatoes, and Feta

Preparation Time: 10 minutes   *Total Time: 15 minutes*   *Servings: 2*

Ingredients:

- 4 large eggs
- 1 cup fresh spinach, chopped
- 1/2 cup cherry tomatoes, halved
- 1/4 cup crumbled feta cheese
- Olive oil for cooking
- Salt and pepper to taste
- Fresh herbs for garnish (optional)

Instructions:

1. In a bowl, beat the eggs and season with salt and pepper.
2. In a pan over medium heat, warm the olive oil.
3. Cook the spinach until it wilts by adding it to the pan along with the cherry tomatoes.
4. Cover the veggies with whisked eggs and wait a little while for them to set.
5. Fold the second half of the omelet over the portion that has feta cheese sprinkled over it.
6. Cook the eggs until they are done.
7. If preferred, garnish this savory Mediterranean Omelette with fresh herbs.

Nutritional Value (Per Serving):

Calories: 280 kcal.	Protein: 16g.	Fat: 20g
Carbohydrates: 8g.	Fiber: 2g.	Sugar: 3g

Whole Grain Pancakes with Fresh Fruit Compote

Preparation Time: 15 minutes   *Total Time: 30 minutes*   *Servings: 2*

Ingredients:

- 1 cup whole wheat flour
- 1 tablespoon baking powder
- 1 tablespoon honey
- 1 cup milk (dairy or plant-based)
- 1 large egg
- Fresh fruit compote (mixed berries, sliced bananas, etc.)
- Maple syrup for drizzling

Instructions:

1. Combine whole wheat flour and baking powder in a bowl.

2. Mix the honey, milk, and egg in another bowl.

3. Stir the wet and dry ingredients together until they are well combined.

4. Turn up the heat to medium on a griddle or nonstick pan.

5. Transfer the batter in sections of 1/4 cup to the griddle and heat it until bubbles appear on top.

6. Cook, flipping once, until golden brown.

7. Drizzle pancakes with maple syrup and top with fresh fruit compote.

Nutritional Value (Per Serving):

Calories: 220 kcal.   Protein: 8g.   Fat: 3g

Carbohydrates: 40g.   Fiber: 6g.   Sugar: 10g

Smoked Salmon and Cream Cheese Bagel with Cucumber

Preparation Time: 10 minutes   *Total Time: 15 minutes*   *Servings: 2*

Ingredients:

- 2 whole grain bagels, sliced and toasted
- 4 oz smoked salmon
- 4 tablespoons cream cheese
- 1 cucumber, thinly sliced
- Fresh dill for garnish
- Lemon wedges for serving

Instructions:

1. Toast the bagel halves and spread cream cheese on them.
2. Top each half of a bagel with smoked salmon.
3. Add cucumber slices on top and sprinkle fresh dill on top.
4. To add even more taste, serve with lemon slices.

Nutritional Value (Per Serving):

Calories: 380 kcal.   Protein: 22g.   Fat: 15g

Carbohydrates: 40g.   Fiber: 8g.   Sugar: 6g

Olive Oil and Herb Scrambled Eggs with Whole Wheat Toast

Preparation Time: 10 minutes　　　　*Total Time: 15 minutes*　　　　*Servings: 2*

Ingredients:

- 4 large eggs
- 2 tablespoons olive oil
- Fresh herbs (such as chives, parsley), chopped
- Salt and pepper to taste
- 4 slices whole wheat bread, toasted

Instructions:

1. Break the eggs into a basin, whisk in the salt and pepper, and season.
2. In a pan over medium heat, warm the olive oil.
3. Add whisked eggs to the pan and keep stirring.
4. As the eggs begin to set, stir in the chopped fresh herbs.
5. Simmer until eggs are just set and have a hint of cream.
6. Top the toasted whole wheat bread with the Herb and Olive Oil Scrambled Eggs.

Nutritional Value (Per Serving):

Calories: 320 kcal.　　　　Protein: 14g.　　　　Fat: 20g

Carbohydrates: 22g.　　　　Fiber: 5g.　　　　Sugar: 2g

Greekstyle Overnight Oats with Honey and Walnuts

Preparation Time: 5 minutes (plus overnight refrigeration)

Total Time: 5 minutes   *Servings: 2*

Ingredients:

- 1 cup rolled oats
- 1 cup Greek yogurt
- 1 cup milk (dairy or plant-based)
- 2 tablespoons honey
- 1/4 cup chopped walnuts
- Fresh berries for topping

Instructions:

1. In a jar or container, combine rolled oats, Greek yogurt, milk, honey, and chopped walnuts.

2. Give it a good stir, cover it, and chill it for the night.

3. Give the mixture a thorough toss in the morning.

4. Before serving these tasty and nourishing Greek-style overnight oats, top with fresh berries.

Nutritional Value (Per Serving):

Calories: 350 kcal

Protein: 18g

Fat: 12g

Carbohydrates: 45g

Fiber: 7g

Sugar: 18g

Mediterranean Breakfast Wrap with Hummus and Vegetables

Preparation Time: 10 minutes   *Total Time: 10 minutes*   *Servings: 2*

Ingredients:

- 2 whole wheat wraps or tortillas
- 1/2 cup hummus
- 1 cup mixed salad greens
- 1/2 cucumber, thinly sliced
- 1 tomato, diced
- Kalamata olives, pitted and sliced
- Feta cheese, crumbled
- Olive oil for drizzling
- Salt and pepper to taste

Instructions:

1. Evenly coat each whole wheat wrap with hummus.
2. Top with cucumber slices, chopped tomatoes, crumbled feta, mixed salad leaves, and olives.
3. Add a drizzle of olive oil and season with salt and pepper.
4. Tightly roll up the wrap by folding the sides.
5. Cut in half and present this colorful Mediterranean Breakfast Wrap.

Nutritional Value (Per Serving):

Calories: 320 kcal.	Protein: 12g.	Fat: 15g
Carbohydrates: 38g.	Fiber: 8g.	Sugar: 4g

Baked Eggs in Tomato and Bell Pepper Cups

Preparation Time: 15 minutes　　　*Total Time: 30 minutes*　　　*Servings: 2*

Ingredients:

- 4 large eggs
- 2 large tomatoes
- 2 bell peppers (any color)
- Olive oil for drizzling
- Fresh herbs (such as basil or parsley), chopped
- Salt and pepper to taste

Instructions:

1. Set oven temperature to 190°C, or 375°F.
2. Remove the caps and hollow out the centers of bell peppers and tomatoes.
3. Arrange the baking sheet with the tomato and bell pepper cups on top.
4. Keeping the yolk whole, crack one egg into each cup.
5. Add salt and pepper to taste and drizzle with olive oil.
6. Continue baking for approximately 1520 minutes, or until the eggs are set to your preference.

Serve these Baked Eggs in Tomato and Bell Pepper Cups with a fresh herb garnish.

Nutritional Value (Per Serving):

Calories: 220 kcal.　　　Protein: 16g　　　Fat: 14g

Carbohydrates: 10g.　　　Fiber: 3g.　　　Sugar: 6g

Chapter 2

Lunch Recipes

Lemon Herb Grilled Chicken Salad

Preparation Time: 15 minutes.   *Servings: 2*

Total Time: 30 minutes (including marination)

Ingredients:

- 2 boneless, skinless chicken breasts
- 1 lemon (zested and juiced)
- 2 tablespoons olive oil
- Fresh herbs (such as rosemary, thyme, or oregano), chopped
- Mixed salad greens
- Cherry tomatoes, halved
- Cucumber, sliced
- Red onion, thinly sliced
- Feta cheese, crumbled
- Salt and pepper to taste

Instructions:

1. Combine the olive oil, chopped herbs, lemon zest, lemon juice, salt, and pepper in a bowl.

2. Let the chicken breasts sit in the mixture for a minimum of fifteen minutes.

3. Cook the chicken completely on the grill.

4. Cut grilled chicken into slices and present it over a bed of mixed salad greens topped with cucumber, red onion, cherry tomatoes, and crumbled feta.

Nutritional Value (Per Serving):

Calories: 400 kcal	Protein: 30g	Fat: 20g
Carbohydrates: 25g	Fiber: 6g	Sugar: 4g

Mediterranean Chickpea and Spinach Stew

Preparation Time: 10 minutes   *Total Time: 25 minutes*   *Servings: 4*

Ingredients:

- 2 cans chickpeas, drained and rinsed
- 1 onion, chopped
- 2 cloves garlic, minced
- 1 can diced tomatoes
- 1 cup vegetable broth
- 1 teaspoon ground cumin
- 1 teaspoon paprika
- 2 cups fresh spinach
- Olive oil for drizzling
- Salt and pepper to taste

Instructions:

1. In a saucepan, soften minced garlic and chopped onion by sautéing them in olive oil.

2. Add chickpeas, diced tomatoes, vegetable broth, ground cumin, paprika, salt, and pepper.

3. Simmer for fifteen minutes.

4. Add the fresh spinach and stir until it wilts.

5. Drizzle this hearty Mediterranean Chickpea and Spinach Stew with olive oil before serving.

Nutritional Value (Per Serving):

Calories: 300 kcal.

Carbohydrates: 45g

Protein: 15g.

Fiber: 12g

Fat: 8g

Sugar: 8g

Quinoa Greek Salad with Cucumber and Feta

Preparation Time: 15 minutes   *Total Time: 25 minutes*   *Servings: 2*

Ingredients:

- 1 cup cooked quinoa
- 1 cucumber, diced
- 1 cup cherry tomatoes, halved
- 1/2 cup feta cheese, crumbled
- Kalamata olives, pitted and sliced
- Red onion, finely chopped
- Fresh parsley, chopped
- Olive oil for dressing
- Lemon juice
- Salt and pepper to taste

Instructions:

1. Put the cooked quinoa, cucumber, cherry tomatoes, feta cheese, olives, red onion, and parsley in a big bowl together.

2. Pour lemon juice and olive oil over the salad.

3. Gently toss to thoroughly combine.

4. Add salt and pepper for seasoning.

5. Offer this energizing Quinoa Greek Salad as a tasty and light meal.

Nutritional Value (Per Serving):

Calories: 320 kcal.   Protein: 10g   Fat: 18g

Carbohydrates: 30g.   Fiber: 5g   Sugar: 3g

Baked Cod with Lemon and Herbs

Preparation Time: 10 minutes   *Total Time: 20 minutes*   *Servings: 2*

Ingredients:

- 2 cod filets
- 1 lemon (zested and sliced)
- Fresh herbs (such as dill or parsley), chopped
- Olive oil for drizzling
- Salt and pepper to taste

Instructions:

1. Set the oven's temperature to 200°C, or 400°F.

2. Arrange the filets of fish on a baking sheet.

3. Add chopped herbs, salt, and pepper for seasoning.

4. Drizzle with olive oil, then arrange lemon slices on top.

5. Bake the fish for 1518 minutes, or until it flakes easily.

6. Accompany this tasty and light-baked cod with a dish of your preferred veggies.

Nutritional Value (Per Serving):

Calories: 250 kcal.   Protein: 30g.   Fat: 12g

Carbohydrates: 2g.   Fiber: 1g.   Sugar: 0g

Lentil and Vegetable Soup with Olive Oil Drizzle

Preparation Time: 15 minutes   *Total Time: 40 minutes*   *Servings: 4*

Ingredients:

- 1 cup dried green or brown lentils
- 1 onion, diced
- 2 carrots, sliced
- 2 celery stalks, chopped
- 2 cloves garlic, minced
- 1 can diced tomatoes
- 6 cups vegetable broth
- 1 teaspoon ground cumin
- 1 teaspoon smoked paprika
- Olive oil for drizzling
- Fresh parsley for garnish
- Salt and pepper to taste

Instructions:

1. Use cold water to rinse the lentils.

2. In a saucepan, soften the celery, carrots, diced onion, and minced garlic by sautéing them in olive oil.

3. Include lentils, smoked paprika, chopped tomatoes, vegetable broth, ground cumin, and salt and pepper.

4. Simmer for twenty-five minutes.

5. Top with fresh parsley and drizzle olive oil over each plate.

Nutritional Value (Per Serving):

Calories: 280 kcal.   Protein: 18g   Fat: 8g

Carbohydrates: 40g.   Fiber: 15g.   Sugar: 5g

Whole Wheat Pita Bread with Hummus and Veggies

Preparation Time: 10 minutes.   *Total Time: 10 minutes.*   *Servings: 2*

Ingredients:

- 4 whole wheat pita bread rounds
- 1 cup hummus
- Cherry tomatoes, halved
- Cucumber, thinly sliced
- Bell peppers, thinly sliced
- Kalamata olives, sliced
- Feta cheese, crumbled
- Fresh herbs (such as mint or parsley), chopped

Instructions:

1. Use an oven or toaster to reheat whole wheat pita bread.

2. Drizzle a thick layer of hummus over each pita.

3. Add crumbled feta, olives, bell pepper, cucumber, and cherry tomato slices on top.

4. Add freshly chopped herbs as a garnish.

Nutritional Value (Per Serving):

Calories: 280 kcal.
Carbohydrates: 35g.

Protein: 10g
Fiber: 8g.

Fat: 12g
Sugar: 2g

Shrimp and Zucchini Skewers with Tzatziki Sauce

Preparation Time: 20 minutes (plus marination time)

Total Time: 30 minutes   *Servings: 4*

Ingredients:

- 1 pound large shrimp, peeled and deveined
- 2 zucchinis, sliced
- Olive oil for marinade
- Lemon juice
- Garlic, minced
- Dried oregano
- Salt and pepper to taste
- Tzatziki sauce for dipping

Instructions:

1. Combine the olive oil, lemon juice, dried oregano, minced garlic, salt, and pepper in a bowl.

2. Let zucchini slices and shrimp marinate in the marinade for at least 20 minutes.

3. Alternately thread zucchini and shrimp onto skewers.

4. Cook the kebabs until the shrimp becomes opaque.

5. Present with a Tzatziki sauce side dish for dipping.

Nutritional Value (Per Serving):

Calories: 220 kcal   Protein: 25g.   Fat: 10g

Carbohydrates: 10g   Fiber: 2g   Sugar: 6g

Eggplant and Tomato Stuffed Peppers

Preparation Time: 20 minutes   *Total Time: 45 minutes*   *Servings: 4*

Ingredients:

- 4 bell peppers, halved and seeds removed
- 1 large eggplant, diced
- 1 onion, chopped
- 2 cloves garlic, minced
- 1 can diced tomatoes
- 1 cup cooked quinoa
- Fresh basil, chopped
- Olive oil for sautéing
- Salt and pepper to taste
- Grated Parmesan cheese for topping

Instructions:

1. Set oven temperature to 190°C, or 375°F.

2. Use olive oil to sauté minced garlic and sliced onion in a skillet until they become tender.

3. Cook until softened after adding the chopped eggplant.

4. Combine cooked quinoa, diced tomatoes, and fresh basil that has been chopped.

5. Add pepper and salt for seasoning.

6. Stuff the eggplant-tomato mixture into bell pepper halves.

7. Top with grated Parmesan cheese.

8. Bake for 25 to 30 minutes, or until the peppers are just soft.

Nutritional Value (Per Serving):

Calories: 300 kcal.	Protein: 8g	Fat: 10g
Carbohydrates: 45g.	Fiber: 10g.	Sugar: 10g

Greek Farro Salad with Cherry Tomatoes and Olives

Preparation Time: 15 minutes   *Total Time: 25 minutes*   *Servings: 2*

Ingredients:

- 1 cup cooked farro
- Cherry tomatoes, halved
- Kalamata olives, sliced
- Red onion, finely chopped
- Cucumber, diced
- Feta cheese, crumbled
- Fresh mint, chopped
- Olive oil for dressing
- Red wine vinegar
- Salt and pepper to taste

Instructions:

1. Put the cooked farro, cherry tomatoes, cucumber, feta cheese, red onion, olives, and chopped mint in a big bowl.

2. Drizzle olive oil and red wine vinegar over the salad.

3. Gently toss to thoroughly combine.

4. Add salt and pepper for seasoning.

5. You can serve this healthy Greek Farro Salad as a delicious main course or as a side dish.

Nutritional Value (Per Serving):

Calories: 280 kcal.   Protein: 8g.   Fat: 10g

Carbohydrates: 40g.   Fiber: 8g.   Sugar: 3g

Spinach and Feta Turkey Burger with Greek Salad

Preparation Time: 20 minutes   *Total Time: 30 minutes*   *Servings: 2*

Ingredients:

For Turkey Burger:

- 1 pound ground turkey
- 1 cup fresh spinach, chopped
- 1/2 cup crumbled feta cheese
- 1 teaspoon dried oregano
- Salt and pepper to taste

For Greek Salad:

- Mixed salad greens
- Cherry tomatoes, halved
- Cucumber, sliced
- Red onion, thinly sliced
- Kalamata olives, sliced
- Feta cheese, crumbled
- Olive oil and lemon juice for dressing
- Salt and pepper to taste

Instructions:

For Turkey Burger:

1. Combine the ground turkey, chopped spinach, feta crumbles, dried oregano, salt, and pepper in a basin.

2. Shape the mixture into patties and cook them on the grill until they are done.

For Greek Salad:

3. Transfer the mixed salad greens, cucumber, red onion, olives, feta cheese, and cherry tomatoes to a different bowl.

4. Add salt and pepper to taste, then drizzle with lemon juice and olive oil.

5. Along with a side of cool Greek salad, serve the Turkey Burger with Spinach and Feta on a whole wheat bun.o

Nutritional Value (Per Serving):

Calories: 350 kcal (burger) + 150 kcal (salad)

Protein: 25g (burger) + 8g (salad)

Fat: 18g (burger) + 12g (salad)

Carbohydrates: 20g (burger) + 15g (salad)

Fiber: 5g (burger) + 4g (salad)

Sugar: 2g (burger) + 5g (salad)

Chapter 3

Dinner Recipes

Grilled Salmon with Lemon and Dill

Preparation Time: 10 minutes (plus marination time)

Total Time: 20 minutes   *Servings: 2*

Ingredients:

- 2 salmon fillets
- 1 lemon (zested and sliced)
- Fresh dill, chopped
- Olive oil for marination
- Salt and pepper to taste

Instructions:

1. Combine olive oil, lemon zest, chopped dill, salt, and pepper in a bowl.
2. For at least half an hour, marinate salmon fillets in the marinade.
3. Grill the fish until it's fully done.
4. Garnish with fresh dill and serve with slices of lemon.

Nutritional Value (Per Serving):

Calories: 300 kcal.   Protein: 25g   Fat: 20g

Carbohydrates: 2g   Fiber: 1g   Sugar: 0g

Mediterranean Baked Chicken with Artichokes and Olives

Preparation Time: 15 minutes   *Total Time: 35 minutes*   *Servings: 2*

Ingredients:

- 2 chicken breasts
- 1 can artichoke hearts, drained and halved
- Kalamata olives, pitted and sliced
- Cherry tomatoes, halved
- Olive oil for drizzling
- Fresh oregano, chopped
- Salt and pepper to taste

Instructions:

1. Set the oven temperature to 190°C, or 375°F.
2. Transfer the chicken breasts to a baking dish.
3. Arrange cherry tomatoes, artichoke hearts, and olives all around the chicken.
4. Drizzle with olive oil and season with salt, pepper, and chopped oregano.
5. Bake until the veggies are soft and the chicken is well cooked.

Nutritional Value (Per Serving):

Calories: 350 kcal.   Protein: 30g.   Fat: 15g

Carbohydrates: 15g   Fiber: 5g.   Sugar: 2g

Quinoa Stuffed Bell Peppers with Ground Turkey

Preparation Time: 20 minutes   *Total Time: 45 minutes*   *Servings: 4*

Ingredients:

- 4 bell peppers, halved and seeds removed
- 1 cup cooked quinoa
- 1/2 pound ground turkey
- Onion, finely chopped
- Garlic, minced
- Tomato sauce
- Italian seasoning
- Salt and pepper to taste
- Shredded mozzarella cheese (optional)

Instructions:

1. Turn the oven on to 375°F, or 190°C.
2. Until softened, sauté minced garlic and diced onion in a skillet.
3. Add the turkey meat and heat it until it browns.
4. Add the tomato sauce, salt, pepper, Italian spice, and cooked quinoa.
5. Stuff the turkey-quinoa mixture into each side of a bell pepper.
6. You may choose to add shredded mozzarella on top.
7. Bake until the cheese has melted and the peppers are soft.

Nutritional Value (Per Serving):

Calories: 300 kcal.   Protein: 20g.   Fat: 10g

Carbohydrates: 30g.   Fiber: 5g.   Sugar: 5g

Eggplant Parmesan with Whole Wheat Pasta

Preparation Time: 30 minutes   *Total Time: 1 hour*   *Servings: 4*

Ingredients:

- 1 large eggplant, sliced
- Whole wheat pasta
- Marinara sauce
- Mozzarella cheese, shredded
- Parmesan cheese, grated
- Fresh basil, chopped
- Olive oil for baking
- Salt and pepper to taste

Instructions:

1. Turn the oven on to 375°F, or 190°C.
2. Season eggplant slices with salt, pepper, and olive oil.
3. Bake in the oven until soft.
4. Arrange cooked whole wheat spaghetti, marinara sauce, cheeses, and pieces of eggplant in a baking dish.
5. Continue layering and add fresh basil on top.
6. Bake till golden and bubbling.

Nutritional Value (Per Serving):

Calories: 400 kcal   Protein: 15g   Fat: 15g

Carbohydrates: 55g   Fiber: 10g.   Sugar: 8g

Greek Lemon Garlic Shrimp with Orzo

Preparation Time: 15 minutes   *Total Time: 25 minutes*   *Servings: 4*

Ingredients:

- 1 pound shrimp, peeled and deveined
- Orzo pasta
- 1 lemon (zested and juiced)
- Garlic, minced
- Olive oil for cooking
- Fresh parsley, chopped
- Salt and pepper to taste

Instructions:

1. Prepare the orzo pasta per the directions on the box.
2. Heat the olive oil in a skillet and fry the minced garlic until it becomes aromatic.
3. Cook the shrimp until they become opaque and pink.
4. Add the zest and juice of the lemon, salt, and pepper.
5. Top cooked orzo with shrimp and sprinkle with fresh parsley.

Nutritional Value (Per Serving):

Calories: 320 kcal   Protein: 25g   Fat: 10g

Carbohydrates: 30g   Fiber: 2g   Sugar: 2g

Baked Cod with Tomato and Olive Relish

Preparation Time: 15 minutes   *Total Time: 30 minutes*   *Servings: 2*

Ingredients:

- 2 cod filets
- Cherry tomatoes, halved
- Kalamata olives, sliced
- Red onion, finely chopped
- Fresh basil, chopped
- Olive oil for drizzling
- Balsamic glaze (optional)
- Salt and pepper to taste

Instructions:

1. Set the oven's temperature to 200°C, or 400°F.
2. Arrange the filets of fish on a baking sheet.
3. Put the chopped red onion, fresh basil, sliced olives, and half of the cherry tomatoes in a bowl.
4. Drizzle the fish with the olive and tomato relish.
5. After the fish is thoroughly cooked, drizzle with olive oil and bake.
6. Before serving, if desired, sprinkle with balsamic glaze.

Nutritional Value (Per Serving):

Calories: 250 kcal   Protein: 30g   Fat: 12g

Carbohydrates: 10g   Fiber: 2g   Sugar: 3g

Lentil and Vegetable StirFry with Brown Rice

Preparation Time: 20 minutes   *Total Time: 30 minutes*   *Servings: 4*

Ingredients:

- 1 cup brown lentils, cooked
- Mixed vegetables (broccoli, bell peppers, carrots), sliced
- Brown rice, cooked
- Soy sauce
- Ginger, minced
- Garlic, minced
- Sesame oil for stirfrying
- Green onions, sliced
- Sesame seeds for garnish

Instructions:

1. Heat the sesame oil in a wok or skillet and fry the minced garlic and ginger.
2. Stir-fry the cut veggies until they are crisp-tender.
3. Add the soy sauce and cooked lentils and stir.
4. Top with sesame seeds and chopped green onions and serve over cooked brown rice.

Nutritional Value (Per Serving):

Calories: 300 kcal   Protein: 15g   Fat: 5g

Carbohydrates: 50g   Fiber: 12g   Sugar: 5g

Greek Chicken Souvlaki Skewers with Tzatziki Sauce

Preparation Time: 15 minutes (plus marination time)

Total Time: 30 minutes   *Servings: 2*

Ingredients:

For Chicken Marinade:

- 1 pound chicken breast, cut into chunks
- Olive oil
- Lemon juice
- Garlic, minced
- Dried oregano
- Salt and pepper to taste

For Tzatziki Sauce:

- Greek yogurt
- Cucumber, grated and drained
- Garlic, minced
- Fresh dill, chopped
- Lemon juice
- Salt and pepper to taste

Instructions:

For Chicken Souvlaki:

1. Combine the olive oil, lemon juice, dried oregano, minced garlic, salt, and pepper in a bowl.

2. Let the chicken pieces marinate in the sauce for a minimum of half an hour.

3. Skewer the marinated chicken and cook it over the grill until it is done.

For Tzatziki Sauce:

4. Grated cucumber, minced garlic, chopped fresh dill, lemon juice, salt, and pepper should all be combined with Greek yogurt in a dish.

5. Provide Tzatziki Sauce on the side for the Chicken Souvlaki skewers.

Nutritional Value (Per Serving):

Calories: 280 kcal (chicken) + 60 kcal (tzatziki)

Protein: 30g (chicken) + 6g (tzatziki)

Fat: 15g (chicken) + 3g (tzatziki)

Carbohydrates: 5g (chicken) + 8g (tzatziki)

Fiber: 1g (chicken) + 1g (tzatziki)

Sugar: 2g (chicken) + 4g (tzatziki)

Spinach and Feta Stuffed Chicken Breast

Preparation Time: 20 minutes   *Total Time: 40 minutes*   *Servings: 2*

Ingredients:

- 2 chicken breasts
- Fresh spinach leaves
- Feta cheese, crumbled
- Garlic, minced
- Olive oil for cooking
- Lemon zest
- Salt and pepper to taste

Instructions:

1. Turn the oven on to 375°F, or 190°C.

2. Give each chicken breast a butterfly wing.

3. Combine fresh spinach leaves, minced garlic, and crumbled feta in a basin.

4. Stuff the spinach and feta mixture into each chicken breast.

5. Add lemon zest, salt, and pepper for seasoning.

6. In an oven-safe skillet with heated olive oil, brown the chicken breasts before transferring them to the oven to complete cooking.

Nutritional Value (Per Serving):

Calories: 320 kcal	Protein: 35g	Fat: 15g
Carbohydrates: 5g	Fiber: 2g	Sugar: 1g

Mediterranean-style Turkey and Vegetable Kebabs

Preparation Time: 20 minutes (plus marination time)

Total Time: 30 minutes   *Servings: 4*

Ingredients:

- 1 pound ground turkey
- Mixed vegetables (bell peppers, cherry tomatoes, red onion), cut into chunks
- Olive oil for marination
- Lemon juice
- Garlic, minced
- Dried oregano
- Salt and pepper to taste

Instructions:

1. Combine ground turkey, dried oregano, lemon juice, olive oil, minced garlic, salt, and pepper in a bowl.

2. Shape the mixture into kebabs and add mixed veggie bits in between.

3. Grill the kebabs until the veggies are soft and the turkey is cooked through.

Nutritional Value (Per Serving):

Calories: 280 kcal　　Protein: 20g　　Fat: 15g

Carbohydrates: 15g　　Fiber: 3g　　Sugar: 5g

Chapter 4

Snacks Recipes

Greek Yogurt and Berry Parfait

Preparation Time: 5 minutes   *Total Time: 5 minutes*   *Servings: 2*

Ingredients:

- Greek yogurt
- Mixed berries (strawberries, blueberries, raspberries)
- Honey
- Granola

Instructions:

1. Arrange granola, mixed berries, and Greek yogurt in a glass or dish.
2. Pour some honey over it.
3. Go through the layers again.
4. Enjoy this cool parfait right away by serving it immediately.

Nutritional Value (Per Serving):

Calories: 250 kcal

Protein: 15g

Fat: 8g

Carbohydrates: 35g

Fiber: 5g

Sugar: 15g

Hummus with Fresh Vegetable Sticks

Preparation Time: 10 minutes   *Total Time: 10 minutes*   *Servings: 4*

Ingredients:

- Hummus
- Carrot sticks
- Cucumber sticks
- Bell pepper strips

Instructions:

1. Fill a serving dish with hummus.
2. Assemble new veggie sticks.
3. Dip the veggie sticks into the hummus.
4. Enjoy this nutritious and enjoyable snack.

Nutritional Value (Per Serving):

Calories: 180 kcal   Protein: 5g   Fat: 10g

Carbohydrates: 20g   Fiber: 6g   Sugar: 5g

Roasted Chickpeas with Mediterranean Spices

Preparation Time: 5 minutes   *Total Time: 30 minutes*   *Servings: 4*

Ingredients:

- Canned chickpeas, drained and rinsed
- Olive oil
- Paprika
- Cumin

- Garlic powder
- Salt

Instructions:

1. Set the oven's temperature to 200°C, or 400°F.
2. Combine chickpeas with salt, garlic powder, cumin, paprika, and olive oil.
3. On a baking sheet arrange the chickpeas
4. Roast until crispy, about 2530 minutes.
5. Let cool, then serve as a crispy snack.

Nutritional Value (Per Serving):

Calories: 180 kcal	Protein: 7g	Fat: 8g
Carbohydrates: 22g	Fiber: 6g	Sugar: 1g

Olive and Feta Cheese Plate

Preparation Time: 5 minutes　　　*Total Time: 5 minutes*　　　*Servings: 2*

Ingredients:

- Kalamata olives
- Green olives
- Feta cheese, cubed
- Extra virgin olive oil
- Fresh oregano (optional)

Instructions:

1. Arrange green olives and Kalamata on a dish.
2. Stir in feta cheese cubes.

3. Add a little extra virgin olive oil drizzle.

4. Garnish with fresh oregano if preferred.

5. As a delicious starter from the Mediterranean.

Nutritional Value (Per Serving):

Calories: 220 kcal

Protein: 8g

Fat: 18g

Carbohydrates: 5g

Fiber: 2g

Sugar: 1g

Whole Wheat Pita with Tzatziki Sauce

Preparation Time: 10 minutes　　*Total Time: 10 minutes*　　*Servings: 2*

Ingredients:

- Whole wheat pita bread
- Tzatziki sauce (Greek yogurt, cucumber, garlic, dill)

Instructions:

1. Warm pita bread made with whole wheat.

2. Accompany with a serving of house-made tzatziki sauce.

3. Dip and savor this traditional Mediterranean finger food.

Nutritional Value (Per Serving):

Calories: 200 kcal

Protein: 8g

Fat: 5g

Carbohydrates: 35g

Fiber: 6g

Sugar: 3g

Caprese Salad Skewers with Balsamic Glaze

Preparation Time: 15 minutes   *Total Time: 15 minutes*   *Servings: 4*

Ingredients:

- Cherry tomatoes
- Fresh mozzarella balls
- Fresh basil leaves
- Balsamic glaze

Instructions:

1. Attach cherry tomatoes, freshly made mozzarella balls, and freshly chopped basil leaves to skewers.

2. Put the kebabs on a plate for serving.

3. Drizzle with balsamic glaze.

4. Serve as a tasty and eye-catching starter.

Nutritional Value (Per Serving):

Calories: 150 kcal

Protein: 8g

Fat: 10g

Carbohydrates: 10g

Fiber: 2g

Sugar: 6g

Almond and Apricot Energy Bites

Preparation Time: 15 minutes

Total Time: 30 minutes

Servings: 8

Ingredients:

- Almonds
- Dried apricots
- Honey
- Rolled oats
- Chia seeds

Instructions:

1. Process almonds, rolled oats, honey, dried apricots, and chia seeds in a food processor until a sticky mixture forms.

2. Create bite-sized balls out of the mixture.

3. Let cool for a minimum of fifteen minutes before to serving.

4. Savor these wholesome, high-energy morsels.

Nutritional Value (Per Serving):

Calories: 180 kcal

Protein: 5g

Fat: 10g

Carbohydrates: 20g

Fiber: 4g

Sugar: 12g

Cucumber and Tomato Bruschetta

Preparation Time: 10 minutes   *Total Time: 15 minutes.*   *Servings: 4*

Ingredients:

- Cucumber, diced
- Cherry tomatoes, diced
- Red onion, finely chopped
- Fresh basil, chopped
- Balsamic vinegar
- Olive oil
- Whole grain baguette slices

Instructions:

1. Combine chopped fresh basil, cherry tomatoes, red onion, and sliced cucumber in a bowl.

2. Use olive oil and balsamic vinegar for drizzling.

3. Place the cucumber and tomato mixture on top of toasted whole grain baguette pieces.

4. Present as a crisp and energizing bruschetta.

Nutritional Value (Per Serving):

Calories: 160 kcal

Protein: 4g

Fat: 5g

Carbohydrates: 25g

Fiber: 4g

Sugar: 5g

Greek-style Spinach and Feta Dip

Preparation Time: 10 minutes

Total Time: 20 minutes

Servings: 6

Ingredients:

- Frozen chopped spinach, thawed and drained
- Greek yogurt
- Feta cheese, crumbled
- Garlic, minced
- Olive oil
- Lemon juice
- Salt and pepper to taste

Instructions:

1. In a bowl, add frozen and drained chopped spinach, Greek yogurt, crumbled feta, minced garlic, olive oil, and lemon juice.
2. Blend until well blended.
3. Add pepper and salt for seasoning.
4. Serve with whole grain pita chips or veggie sticks.

Nutritional Value (Per Serving):

Calories: 160 kcal

Protein: 8g

Fat: 12g

Carbohydrates: 6g

Fiber: 2g

Sugar: 2g

Baked Zucchini Chips with Herbs

Preparation Time: 15 minutes   *Total Time: 25 minutes*   *Servings: 4*

Ingredients:

- Zucchini, thinly sliced
- Olive oil
- Dried herbs (rosemary, thyme, oregano)
- Parmesan cheese, grated
- Salt and pepper to taste

Instructions:

1. Set the oven temperature to 190°C, or 375°F.
2. Toss thinly sliced zucchini with olive oil, dried herbs, grated Parmesan cheese, salt, and pepper.
3. Put in order on a baking sheet.
4. Bake until crispy and golden.
5. Act as a guilt-free alternative for regular chips.

Nutritional Value (Per Serving):

Calories: 120 kcal

Protein: 3g

Fat: 8g

Carbohydrates: 10g

Fiber: 3g

Sugar: 5g

Chapter 5

Dessert Recipes

Greek Yogurt and Honey Panna Cotta

Preparation Time: 15 minutes   *Servings: 4*

Total Time: 4 hours (including chilling time)

Ingredients:

- 2 cups Greek yogurt
- 1/2 cup honey
- 2 teaspoons gelatin
- 1/4 cup water
- Vanilla extract (optional)

Instructions:

1. Combine Greek yogurt and honey in a dish.
2. Bloom the gelatin in water in a separate basin.
3. Bring the gelatin mixture to a full boil and dissolve.
4. Mix the yogurt-honey combination with the gelatin mixture.
5. Fill molds, then chill until solid.

Nutritional Value (Per Serving):

Calories: 200 kcal

Protein: 15g

Fat: 6g

Carbohydrates: 25g

Fiber: 0g

Sugar: 22g

Almond and Orange Flourless Cake

Preparation Time: 15 minutes   *Total Time: 45 minutes*   *Servings: 8*

Ingredients:

- 2 cups almond flour
- 4 eggs
- 1/2 cup honey
- Zest and juice of 2 oranges
- Baking powder
- Vanilla extract

Instructions:

1. Set the oven's temperature to 175°C/350°F.
2. Combine almond flour, eggs, honey, orange juice, zest, baking powder, and vanilla essence in a bowl.
3. Transfer the batter to a cake pan that has been oiled.
4. Bake for a whole toothpick's duration.

Nutritional Value (Per Serving):

Calories: 250 kcal

Protein: 8g

Fat: 18g

Carbohydrates: 20g

Fiber: 4g

Sugar: 14g

Poached Pears in Red Wine Reduction

Preparation Time: 15 minutes   *Total Time: 1 hour*   *Servings: 4*

Ingredients:

- 4 ripe pears, peeled and halved
- 1 bottle red wine
- 1 cup sugar
- 1 cinnamon stick
- 4 cloves
- Vanilla bean (optional)

Instructions:

1. Put the sugar, vanilla bean, cinnamon stick, cloves, and red wine in a saucepan.
2. Include the peeled and cut pears.
3. Simmer the pears until they are soft.
4. Drizzle the red wine reduction over top before serving.

Nutritional Value (Per Serving):

Calories: 180 kcal

Protein: 1g

Fat: 0g

Carbohydrates: 40g

Fiber: 4g

Sugar: 32g

Olive Oil and Lemon Cake

Preparation Time: 20 minutes　　　*Total Time: 1 hour*　　　*Servings: 10*

Ingredients:

- 2 cups all purpose flour
- 1 cup olive oil
- 1 cup sugar
- 4 eggs
- Zest and juice of 2 lemons
- Baking powder
- Vanilla extract

Instructions:

1. Set the oven temperature to 175°C, or 350°F.

2. Combine flour, sugar, eggs, lemon zest, lemon juice, baking powder, and vanilla essence in a bowl.

3. Transfer the mixture onto a cake pan that has been coated with oil.

4. Bake for a toothpick to come out clean.

Nutritional Value (Per Serving):

Calories: 280 kcal

Protein: 4g

Fat: 18g

Carbohydrates: 26g

Fiber: 1g

Sugar: 14g

Yogurt and Berry Frozen Popsicles

Preparation Time: 10 minutes

Total Time: 4 hours (including freezing time)

Servings: 6

Ingredients:

- 2 cups Greek yogurt
- Mixed berries (strawberries, blueberries, raspberries)
- Honey

Instructions:

1. Combine Greek yogurt and honey in a dish.
2. Line popsicle molds with a layer of yogurt and mixed berries.
3. After inserting the popsicle sticks, freeze until firm.

Nutritional Value (Per Serving):

Calories: 120 kcal

Protein: 8g

Fat: 2g

Carbohydrates: 20g

Fiber: 2g

Sugar: 15g

Fig and Walnut Biscotti

Preparation Time: 15 minutes   *Total Time: 1 hour and 15 minutes*   *Servings: 12*

Ingredients:
- 2 cups all-purpose flour
- 1 cup sugar
- 3 eggs
- 1 cup dried figs, chopped
- 1 cup walnuts, chopped
- Baking powder
- Vanilla extract

Instructions:
1. Set the oven's temperature to 175°C/350°F.
2. Combine the flour, sugar, eggs, baking powder, vanilla essence, chopped walnuts, and figs in a bowl.
3. Onto a baking sheet, shape the dough into a log.
4. Slice into biscotti shapes after baking till brown.
5. Continue baking until crisp.

Nutritional Value (Per Serving):
Calories: 180 kcal

Protein: 4g

Fat: 8g

Carbohydrates: 25g

Fiber: 2g

Sugar: 12g

Pistachio and Honey Baklava

Preparation Time: 30 minutes   *Total Time: 1 hour and 30 minutes*   *Servings: 20*

Ingredients:

- Phyllo pastry sheets
- 2 cups pistachios, chopped
- 1 cup unsalted butter, melted
- 1 cup honey
- Cinnamon
- Cloves

Instructions:

1. Set the oven temperature to 175°C, or 350°F.
2. Place sheets of phyllo pastry in a baking dish after brushing them with melted butter.
3. Combine chopped pistachios with cloves and cinnamon.
4. Top the phyllo layers with a sprinkle of the pistachio mixture.
5. Continue layering, then bake until brown.
6. Drizzle honey on top of the cooked baklava.

Nutritional Value (Per Serving):

Calories: 300 kcal

Protein: 5g

Fat: 20g

Carbohydrates: 30g

Fiber: 2g

Sugar: 15g

Orange and Date Salad with Mint

Preparation Time: 10 minutes   *Total Time: 10 minutes*   *Servings: 4*

Ingredients:

- Oranges, peeled and sliced
- Dates, pitted and chopped
- Fresh mint leaves
- Orange juice
- Honey

Instructions:

1. Arrange the orange slices on a dish for serving.
2. Top the oranges with sliced dates.
3. Add a honey and orange juice drizzle.
4. Add some mint leaves as a garnish.

Nutritional Value (Per Serving):

Calories: 120 kcal

Protein: 1g

Fat: 0g

Carbohydrates: 30g

Fiber: 4g

Sugar: 24g

Chia Seed Pudding with Mediterranean Fruit

Preparation Time: 10 minutes (plus chilling time)

Total Time: 4 hours   *Servings: 2*

Ingredients:

1/2 cup chia seeds

2 cups almond milk

1 teaspoon vanilla extract

Mixed Mediterranean fruits (figs, pomegranate seeds, kiwi)

Instructions:

1. Stir the almond milk, vanilla essence, and chia seeds together in a bowl.

2. Let the mixture thicken by refrigerating it.

3. Arrange assorted Mediterranean fruits on top of the chia pudding layer.

4. Serve cold.

Nutritional Value (Per Serving):

Calories: 180 kcal

Protein: 5g

Fat: 10g

Carbohydrates: 20g

Fiber: 8g

Sugar: 8g

Roasted Peaches with Greek Yogurt and Cinnamon

Preparation Time: 15 minutes   *Total Time: 30 minutes*   *Servings: 4*

Ingredients:

- Peaches, halved and pitted
- Greek yogurt
- Honey
- Cinnamon

Instructions:

1. Turn the oven on to 375°F, or 190°C.

2. Put each half of the peach on a baking sheet.

3. Simmer until softened over medium heat.

4. Garnish with a cinnamon sprinkle, a honey drizzle, and a dollop of Greek yogurt.

Nutritional Value (Per Serving):

Calories: 150 kcal

Protein: 8g

Fat: 2g

Carbohydrates: 30g

Fiber: 4g

Sugar: 26g

Conclusion

To sum up, implementing a Mediterranean diet for chronic kidney disease presents a tasty and varied gastronomic experience as well as a proactive measure to promote kidney health. Through the use of basic ingredients, health-conscious cooking methods, and a range of recipes designed for various mealtimes, this cookbook seeks to empower people on their path to the best possible renal health. This integrated approach integrates the Mediterranean diet with mindfulness to create a sustainable and joyful way of living, including fitness choices influenced by the area. I hope that these dishes and ideas may improve the health of those dealing with chronic renal illness in addition to pleasing palates.

Bonus 1

Easy 5 Mediterranean Friendly Exercises for Kidney Health

1. Mediterranean-Inspired Yoga: Incorporate soft, flowing motions into your yoga sessions to embrace the peacefulness of the Mediterranean lifestyle. These sessions are inspired by the region's beautiful scenery.

2. running or Walking Along the Seafront: Move your workout outside by running or walking along the waterfront. The refreshing aspect of the Mediterranean atmosphere is included in your cardio exercise regimen.

3. Dance to Mediterranean Beats: Infuse your exercise with excitement by dancing to Mediterranean music. Dancing, whether to contemporary rhythms or traditional folk dances, is a fun and vivacious way to be active.

4. Riding Outside on Scenic Routes: Take a bike ride through scenic landscapes to discover the beauty of the Mediterranean surroundings. This low-impact workout improves cardiovascular health and is visually pleasing.

5. Water Aerobics Inspired by the Mediterranean: If you have access to a pool, try out some water aerobics that have moves modeled by the Mediterranean's fluidity. This easy, low-impact exercise is great for sore joints and provides a good workout.

Bonus 2

14 Day Meal Plan

Day 1:

Breakfast: Greek Yogurt Parfait with Berries and Almonds

Lunch: Mediterranean Chickpea and Spinach Stew

Dinner: Grilled Salmon with Lemon and Dill

Snack: Hummus with Fresh Vegetable Sticks

Day 2:

Breakfast: Quinoa Breakfast Bowl with Spinach and Poached Egg

Lunch: Lentil and Vegetable StirFry with Brown Rice

Dinner: Mediterranean Baked Chicken with Artichokes and Olives

Snack: Olive and Feta Cheese Plate

Day 3:

Breakfast: Whole Grain Pancakes with Fresh Fruit Compote

Lunch: Eggplant Parmesan with Whole Wheat Pasta

Dinner: Quinoa Stuffed Bell Peppers with Ground Turkey

Snack: Roasted Chickpeas with Mediterranean Spices

Day 4:

Breakfast: Mediterranean Avocado Toast with Tomato and Feta

Lunch: Greek Lemon Garlic Shrimp with Orzo

Dinner: Baked Cod with Lemon and Herbs

Snack: Greek Yogurt and Berry Parfait

Day 5:

Breakfast: Baked Eggs in Tomato and Bell Pepper Cups

Lunch: Spinach and Feta Stuffed Chicken Breast

Dinner: Eggplant and Tomato Stuffed Peppers

Snack: Almond and Apricot Energy Bites

Day 6:

Breakfast: Greekstyle Overnight Oats with Honey and Walnuts

Lunch: Whole Wheat Pita Bread with Hummus and Veggies

Dinner: Shrimp and Zucchini Skewers with Tzatziki Sauce

Snack: Caprese Salad Skewers with Balsamic Glaze

Day 7:

Breakfast: Olive Oil and Herb Scrambled Eggs with Whole Wheat Toast

Lunch: Quinoa Greek Salad with Cucumber and Feta

Dinner: Mediterraneanstyle Turkey and Vegetable Kebabs

Snack: Greek-style Spinach and Feta Dip

Day 8:

Breakfast: Greek Yogurt Parfait with Berries and Almonds

Lunch: Mediterranean Chickpea and Spinach Stew

Dinner: Grilled Salmon with Lemon and Dill

Snack: Hummus with Fresh Vegetable Sticks

Day 9:

Breakfast: Quinoa Breakfast Bowl with Spinach and Poached Egg
Lunch: Lentil and Vegetable StirFry with Brown Rice
Dinner: Mediterranean Baked Chicken with Artichokes and Olives
Snack: Olive and Feta Cheese Plate

Day 10:

Breakfast: Whole Grain Pancakes with Fresh Fruit Compote

Lunch: Eggplant Parmesan with Whole Wheat Pasta

Dinner: Quinoa Stuffed Bell Peppers with Ground Turkey

Snack: Roasted Chickpeas with Mediterranean Spices

Day 11:

Breakfast: Mediterranean Avocado Toast with Tomato and Feta

Lunch: Greek Lemon Garlic Shrimp with Orzo

Dinner: Baked Cod with Lemon and Herbs

Snack: Greek Yogurt and Berry Parfait

Day 12:

Breakfast: Baked Eggs in Tomato and Bell Pepper Cups

Lunch: Spinach and Feta Stuffed Chicken Breast

Dinner: Eggplant and Tomato Stuffed Peppers

Snack: Almond and Apricot Energy Bites

Day 13:

Breakfast: Greekstyle Overnight Oats with Honey and Walnuts

Lunch: Whole Wheat Pita Bread with Hummus and Veggies

Dinner: Shrimp and Zucchini Skewers with Tzatziki Sauce

Snack: Caprese Salad Skewers with Balsamic Glaze

Day 14:

Breakfast: Olive Oil and Herb Scrambled Eggs with Whole Wheat Toast
Lunch: Quinoa Greek Salad with Cucumber and Feta
Dinner: Mediterraneanstyle Turkey and Vegetable Kebabs
Snack: Greek-style Spinach and Feta Dip

Dear Reader,

I trust you've found our cookbook, tailored for those with chronic kidney disease, to be a flavorful journey through the Mediterranean culinary landscape. Your feedback is invaluable to us, and we would be truly grateful if you could spare a moment to share your thoughts. Your review not only helps us enhance our content but also assists fellow readers in making informed choices.

Thank you for being part of our culinary exploration, and we eagerly anticipate hearing your insights.

Warm regards,

Cynthia P. Allison
Author, Mediterranean Diet Cookbook for Chronic Kidney Disease

www.ingramcontent.com/pod-product-compliance
Lightning Source LLC
Chambersburg PA
CBHW080940260726
48661CB00010B/4018